The #2022 Keto Diet Book

Quick and Healthy Keto
Recipes incl. Breakfast, Lunch,
Dinner, Snacks & More

Morgan Parkins

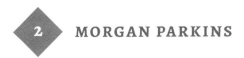 MORGAN PARKINS

TABLE OF CONTENTS

INTRODUCTION

The ketogenic diet (or Keto, for short) is a low carbohydrate, high fat diet that offers a range of health benefits. In fact, this type of diet can help you to lose weight and improve your overall health.

At first, the concept of starting a Keto diet might be daunting, however it does not need to be as complicated as it might sound. Throughout this book, we will explain the basics of the Keto diet, and give you a variety of recipes that will enable you to still enjoy satisfying, filling meals.

Keto Basics

In simple terms, the ketogenic diet is a very low carbohydrate, high fat diet. This diet involves dramatically reducing carbohydrate intake, and replacing it with fat. The dramatic reduction in carbohydrate intake puts your body into ketosis.

Usually, the body creates energy from carbohydrates and glucose. When the body is in ketosis, the body becomes more efficient at burning fat for energy, and stops needing to use carbohydrates. The liver also turns fat into ketones, which can supply energy to the brain.

The Keto diet works by excluding high-carbohydrate foods such as starchy fruits and vegetables, bread, grains, pasta, and sugar, whilst increasing intake of high-fat foods, such as cream, butter, and nuts.

Origins of the Keto Diet and Epilepsy

In medicine, the ketogenic diet is most used to treat hard-to-control epilepsy in children, and was first developed for this purpose in the 1920s. This method of treating refractory epilepsy in children was popular in the 1920s and 1930s until new, successful anticonvulsant drugs began to become available.

The use of the ketogenic diet for treating epilepsy declined further in the 1970s following the introduction of new anticonvulsants such as sodium valproate.

Even today, around 25% to 30% of individuals are unable to control their epilepsy with medication. For this group of patients, in particular the children, the ketogenic diet is sometimes still used as part of a treatment plan.

In addition to treating epilepsy, the ketogenic diet has also been studied for potential use in treating various other neurological disorders, such as headaches, pain, sleep disorders, neurotrauma, and more.

Side Effects of the Ketogenic Diet

A common side effect (albeit a temporary one) of following a ketogenic diet is known as "keto flu". This is the stage during which your body is adjusting to the change in diet. It can cause a variety of symptoms, such as headaches, nausea, and constipation. This usually passes within a couple of weeks, but a registered dietitian will be able to help you minimise them.

Types of Keto Diet

There are several variations of the Keto diet that you can choose from, depending on your health and wellbeing goals. These include:

Standard Ketogenic Diet

The standard Keto diet is a very low carbohydrate diet, with moderate protein and high fat intake. This diet typically contains 70% fat, 20% protein, and only 10% carbohydrates.

Cyclical Ketogenic Diet

The cyclical Keto diet involves periods of high carbohydrate intake and periods of low carbohydrate intake. For example, 5 ketogenic days followed by 2 high carbohydrate days.

Targeted Ketogenic Diet

The targeted ketogenic diet allows you the flexibility of eating extra carbohydrates around workouts.

High Protein Ketogenic Diet

The high protein variation is like the standard ketogenic diet, but includes more protein. The ratio for the high protein ketogenic diet is often 60% fat, 35% protein, and 5% carbohydrates.

However, it is worth bearing in mind that only the standard and high protein diet variations have been studied extensively for their benefits and pitfalls. The cyclical and targeted variations are advanced ketogenic diets that are primarily used by athletes or bodybuilders.

What is Ketosis?

Ketosis is the metabolic state in which the body burns fat instead of carbohydrates for fuel. This state occurs when you drastically reduce the amount of carbohydrates you eat, limiting the body's supply of glucose.

A ketogenic diet is the most effective way to enter ketosis. This requires limiting your carbohydrate consumption to between 20 and 50 grams a day, and replacing the difference with fats, such as meat, fish, eggs, and nuts.

If you are chasing ketosis, it is also important to moderate protein consumption. In high amounts, protein can be converted into glucose, which can slow the transition into ketosis.

Ketoacidosis

Whilst a healthy, low-carbohydrate diet shouldn't cause a problem, it is important to be aware of the symptoms of ketoacidosis.

If you have diabetes that is not under control, a build-up of ketones because of ketosis can become dangerous. High levels can lead to dehydration and change the chemical balance of your blood. This is known as ketoacidosis, or diabetic ketoacidosis. Diabetic ketoacidosis can also occur if people with diabetes do not get enough insulin, or don't drink enough fluids.

Ketoacidosis can also be caused by alcoholism, starvation, or an overactive thyroid.

If you develop any of the following symptoms, call a doctor:

- Thirstiness or a dry mouth
- Peeing a lot
- Extreme tiredness
- Dry, or flushed skin
- Upset stomach or throwing up
- Trouble breathing
- Confusion
- Fruity-smelling breath

Keto for Weight Loss

Following a ketogenic diet is an effective method of weight loss, and it can help lower risk factors for some diseases and conditions. In fact, studies have shown that when compared to other diets, low-carbohydrate and Keto diets can lead to greater weight loss.

By cutting the amount of carbohydrates you eat and replacing them with fat, your overall level of calories eaten should reduce, which will help you lose weight.

The restrictions and requirements of a Keto diet also can naturally help you eat less, because you will start to feel more satisfied at the end of mealtimes.

Health Benefits

In addition to losing weight, the Keto diet can have benefits for some conditions, including diabetes, neurological conditions, and more.

Diabetes

When it comes to managing both diabetes and prediabetes, the Keto diet can improve insulin sensitivity and provide a boost to blood sugar management. Following this type of diet can also help burn excess fat, which is closely linked to type 2 diabetes and prediabetes.

Heart Disease

Following a ketogenic diet can improve risk factors for heart disease such as high blood sugar, high blood pressure, and body fat.

Epilepsy

Research has shown that following a ketogenic diet can cause a reduction in seizures in children with some types of epilepsy.

Acne

Some evidence shows that there is a link between acne and carbohydrates, so cutting down on them can help ease acne. It is also possible that the drop in insulin levels caused by eating a ketogenic diet can help stop breakouts.

Research into the benefits of a ketogenic diet is still ongoing, and more information is becoming available regularly. If you are considering starting a Keto diet to manage a condition, consult your doctor or health professional beforehand to make sure it is right for you.

Food Guide

When planning a Keto diet, you should try to base most of your meals around meat, fatty fish, eggs, dairy, unprocessed cheese, nuts, healthy oils, avocados, and low carbohydrate vegetables, however there are exceptions to certain food groups that do apply.

Protein

Keto diets aren't generally high in protein as they focus on fat, so these should all be consumed in moderation. Eggs, grass-fed beef, fatty fish (such as salmon), and the dark meat chicken are all good sources of protein for a ketogenic diet.

An egg, for example, contains 77 calories, 1g carbohydrates, 6g protein, and 5g fat.

On occasion, proteins such as bacon, and low-fat proteins like skinless chicken and shrimp are acceptable.

You should try to avoid cold cuts of meat that have added sugar, meat that has been marinated in sugary sauces, and processed meat, such as fish or chicken nuggets.

Oils and Fats

When it comes to added oils and fats, avocado, olive, and coconut oil are all suitable choices. In addition, you can also use butter and heavy cream.

As an example of a keto-friendly oil, a tablespoon of avocado oil contains no carbohydrates, no protein, 14g of fat, and 124 calories.

On occasion, you can consume sunflower and corn oils. You should, however, avoid margarine and artificial trans fats.

Fruit and Vegetables

Avocados, leafy greens, celery, and asparagus can all be consumed liberally within a ketogenic diet. Leeks, spaghetti squash, and aubergine can all be eaten occasionally, but you will need to count the carbohydrates.

Half an avocado, for example, contains 160 calories, 2g carbohydrates, 2g protein, and 15g of fat. Avocado is also packed with fibre, which is something that you may find you lack when following a ketogenic diet.

You should avoid potatoes, corn, and raisins.

Nuts and Seeds

Walnuts, almonds, flaxseed, and chia seeds can all be consumed liberally as part of a ketogenic diet. On occasion, you can enjoy cashews, pistachios, and unsweetened nut butters.

You should avoid trail mixes with dried fruit, sweetened nut or seed butters, and chocolate covered nuts.

Dairy Products

You can liberally enjoy cheddar, blue, and feta cheeses, and occasionally enjoy full-fat cottage cheese, Greek yoghurt, and ricotta cheese.

Cheddar cheese, for example, typically contains no carbs, 7g of protein, 9g of fat, and 113 calories per slice.

You should avoid milk, sweetened low-fat yoghurt, and ice creams that aren't keto-friendly.

Drinks

You can liberally enjoy water, almond milk, bone broth, and plain tea as part of a ketogenic diet. On occasion, you can have black coffee (but watch your caffeine consumption), unsweetened carbonated water, diet fizzy drinks, and zero-calorie drinks.

You should avoid sugary fizzy drinks, fruit juices, and lemonade.

Foods to Avoid

When sticking to a keto diet, all food that is high in carbohydrates should be limited. This includes:

- Sugary foods, such as soda, fruit juice, smoothies, ice cream, candy, cake, etc
- Grains and starches, such as wheat, rice, cereal, and pasta
- All fruits, except small portions of berries, like strawberries
- Beans or legumes, such as peas, kidney beans, chickpeas, or lentils
- Root vegetables and tubers, such as potatoes, sweet potatoes, parsnips, and carrots
- Low fat or diet alternatives, such as low-fat mayonnaise, salad dressings, and condiments
- Certain condiments and sauces, such as barbecue sauce, teriyaki, honey mustard, and ketchup
- Unhealthy fats, such as processed vegetable oils and mayonnaise

Common Mistakes

The exact approach to a Keto diet will vary depending on the person. To achieve success, however, there are some common mistakes that should be avoided to achieve success.

Eating Too Much Fat

A common misconception is that fat is a "free food" on a keto diet. Whilst you should be eating more fat on a Keto diet, that doesn't mean that you can eat as much of it as you want, especially if you are trying to lose weight.

Eating Too Much Dairy and Too Many Nuts

Whilst most nuts and some dairy products are Keto friendly, they should be consumed in small, controlled portions. If you eat too much of these food groups, their carbohydrates and calories can easily add up.

Avoiding Protein

A common concern is that eating too much protein when following a Keto diet will lead to gluconeogenesis (your body making new glucose). However, this concern is generally unfounded. Studies in people with type 2 diabetes have suggested that it has little to no effect on blood sugar levels. If you are concerned about your blood sugar, speak to your doctor or nurse.

RECIPES

It is much easier to eat well when sticking to a Keto diet than you might think! In this section, you will find a range of Keto-friendly recipes for breakfast, lunch, dinner, dessert, and snacks.

We've included a range of recipes containing meat and others that are vegetarian, and many of the recipes can be easily adapted to suit different dietary requirements and tastes.

BREAKFAST

Following a Keto diet doesn't need to mean that you scrimp on breakfast. Our breakfast keto recipes are all wholesome and easy to make, perfect for busy mornings.

The key to whipping up a breakfast that is Keto friendly is keeping your kitchen stocked with a few staple ingredients, such as eggs, avocados, bacon, cheese, and your favourite cold cuts of meat or ready to eat fish.

Fluffy Scrambled Eggs

Serves 2
Per serving: 141 calories, 12.1g protein, 2.1g carbohydrates, 9.3g fat

Ingredients

- 4 eggs
- 60ml // ¼ cup milk
- ¼ tsp salt

Instructions

1 Crack the eggs into a microwave-proof bowl. Add the milk and salt, then mix well.

2 Microwave the eggs on high power for 30 seconds.

3 Remove the bowl, beat the eggs well, and scrape down the sides of the bowl. Return to the microwave for another 30 seconds.

4 Repeat this pattern, stirring every 30 seconds for up to 2 ½ minutes.

5 Stop when eggs are cooked to the consistency you desire.

Green Eggs

Serves 2
Per serving: 298 calories, 18g protein, 8g carbohydrates, 18g fat

Ingredients

- 1½ tbsp rapeseed oil
- 2 trimmed and sliced leeks
- 2 garlic cloves, sliced
- ½ tsp coriander seeds
- ½ tsp fennel seeds
- Pinch of chilli flakes, plus extra to serve
- 200g // 7oz spinach
- 2 eggs
- 2 tbsp Greek yogurt
- Squeeze of lemon

Instructions

1 Heat the oil in a large frying pan. Add the leeks and a pinch of salt, then cook until soft.

2 Add the garlic, coriander, fennel, and chilli flakes. Once the seeds begin to crackle, tip in the spinach, and turn down the heat.

3 Stir everything together until the spinach has wilted and reduced, then scrape it over to one side of the pan.

4 Pour a little oil into the pan, then crack in the eggs and fry until cooked to your liking.

5 Stir the yogurt through the spinach mix and season. Top with the fried egg, squeeze over a little lemon and season with black pepper and chilli flakes to serve.

Tomato Baked Eggs

Serves 4
Per serving: 204 calories, 9g protein, 7g carbohydrates, 16g fat

Ingredients

- 900g // 31oz tomatoes
- 3 garlic cloves
- 3 tbsp olive oil
- 4 large eggs
- 2 tbsp chopped parsley

Instructions

1   Preheat the oven to 180C // 350F. Chop the tomatoes into quarters, then put in a shallow ovenproof dish.

2   Peel and slice the garlic before adding to the tomatoes. Drizzle with the oil, season to taste and stir together.

3   Bake for 40 minutes until the tomatoes are softened and starting to brown.

4   Make four wells in the tomato mixture. Crack an egg into each gap and cover the tray with foil. Bake for 5-10 minutes or until the eggs are cooked.

5   Scatter with the herbs and serve piping hot.

Bacon and Egg Baked Avocado

Serves 1
Per serving: 254 calories, 8g protein, 8g carbohydrates, 21g fat

Ingredients

- 1 large avocado
- 2 medium eggs
- 2 tbsp chopped bacon
- Some chives to snip on top (optional)

Instructions

1 Pre-heat the oven to 220C // 425F.
2 Slice the avocados in half, and remove the stones, trying to keep the indent left from the pit as intact as possible.
3 Crack an egg into each avocado.
4 Top the egg with desired amount of chopped bacon.
5 Place in the oven and bake for 15 minutes or until the egg reaches your desired consistency.
6 Remove from the oven and serve immediately.

1 Minute Mug Muffins

Serves 1
Per serving: 322 calories, 18g protein, 4g carbohydrates, 25g fat

Ingredients

- 2 tsp butter or coconut oil
- 2 eggs
- 4 tsp coconut flour
- 1 tsp baking powder
- 1 pinch salt
- 4 tbsp crumbled feta cheese, or grated cheddar cheese
- 2 tbsp fresh basil, chopped

Instructions

1 Grease a ramekin or large mug with the butter or oil.
2 Combine the egg, coconut flour, baking powder, and salt in a bowl. Mix well with a whisk or fork. Allow the batter to thicken for a couple of minutes.
3 Add the feta cheese and basil, then stir until combined.
4 Spoon the batter into the ramekins or microwave-safe mugs. Cook in the microwave on high for 45 seconds to one minute. Alternatively, these can be baked in the oven, at 200C // 400F for 12 minutes.
5 Let the muffins cool for a few minutes before eating.

Breakfast Wrap

Serves 1
Per serving: 552 calories, 28g protein, 5g carbohydrates, 46g fat

Ingredients

- 28g // 1oz bacon
- 2 eggs
- 2 tbsp full-fat milk
- ½ tsp chilli powder
- ½ tbsp fresh chives
- Salt and pepper to season
- 1 tbsp butter
- ¼ avocado, diced
- 3 tbsp mozzarella, shredded
- 1 tbsp sour cream

Instructions

1 Fry the bacon in a large frying pan over medium heat, for 10 minutes or until crispy. Place the bacon on paper towels to absorb any excess fat.
2 Once cooled, chop into small pieces and set aside.
3 Whisk the eggs, cream, chili powder, chives, salt, and pepper in a small bowl.
4 Melt the butter in the frying pan, then pour in the egg mixture.
5 Swirl the frying pan until the egg mixture is evenly spread and thin. This will act as the wrap for your filling.
6 Place a lid over the egg 'wrap' and leave to cook for 2 minutes.
7 Gently lift the 'wrap from the frying pan with a clean spatula onto a plate.
8 Add the mozzarella cheese, bacon, avocado, and sour cream to the egg wrap, then fold the wrap and serve.

High Protein Breakfast Bowl

Serves 1
Per serving: 373 calories, 33g protein, 5g carbohydrates, 24g fat

Ingredients

- 2 large boiled eggs, cut in half
- 100g // 3½oz smoked or cured salmon
- 85g // 3oz cucumber, diced or cut into ribbons
- 2 tbsp cream cheese
- ½ tsp dried chives (optional)
- ¼ lemon (optional)

Instructions

Arrange everything in a bowl. Sprinkle the chives on top if using, or season with salt and pepper to taste.

Spicy Green Omelette

Serves 1
Per serving: 373 calories, 33g protein, 5g carbohydrates, 24g fat

Ingredients

- 2 large eggs
- 2 tbsp finely chopped fresh cilantro or parsley
- 2 tbsp whipping cream
- 1 green chilli, deseeded and sliced
- 1 tbsp butter
- 28g // 1oz grated cheddar cheese
- 35g // 1¼oz watercress or baby spinach
- Salt and pepper to season

Instructions

1 Crack the eggs into a bowl, and add the herbs, cream, and green chilli.
2 Whisk with a fork until well combined. Season with plenty of black pepper and a pinch of salt. Set aside.
3 Melt the butter in a small, non-stick frying pan over a medium heat. Add the egg mixture. Use a spatula to move the eggs around for about a minute while they cook.
4 When the outer edges become opaque, run the spatula around the rim of the pan to loosen it. Shake the pan to make sure the omelette can slide.
5 Scatter cheese over the entire omelette, followed by the watercress. Reduce the heat to low, cover, and leave to cook for a couple of minutes. Serve piping hot.

Turkey and Avocado Plate

Serves 2
Per serving: 525 calories, 26g protein, 7g carbohydrates, 43g fat

Ingredients

- 230g // 8oz cooked turkey
- 1 avocado, sliced
- 35g // 1¼oz lettuce
- 55g // 2oz cream cheese
- 2 tbsp olive oil
- Salt and pepper to taste

Instructions

1. Place an equal amount of turkey, avocado, lettuce, and cream cheese on each plate.
2. Drizzle olive oil over the vegetables and season to taste with salt and pepper.

Scrambled Eggs, Spinach and Smoked Salmon

Serves 1
Per serving: 419 calories, 25g protein, 2g carbohydrates, 34g fat

Ingredients

- 1 tbsp butter
- 2 tbsp whipping cream
- 2 large eggs
- Salt and pepper
- 28g // 1oz baby spinach
- 55g // 2oz smoked salmon

Instructions

1 Heat the butter in a frying pan. Add the baby spinach and cook until soft.
2 Add the cream and let it bubble for a couple of seconds until creamy.
3 Crack the eggs straight into the pan and stir to incorporate.
4 Season with salt and pepper. Keep stirring the mixture until it's cooked to your preference.
5 Put the scrambled eggs on a plate and serve them together with smoked salmon.

TOP TIP

If you aren't a fan of salmon, try it with bacon instead!

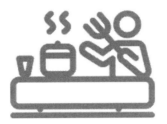

LUNCH

Our Keto lunch recipes are all full of healthy ingredients that are easy to find at your local supermarket or grocery store. Some of these meals can easily be made in advance as part of a meal prep plan, and others can be adapted to make use of leftover meat or vegetables.

Mediterranean Sardine Salad

Serves 4
Per serving: 140 calories, 10g protein, 1g carbohydrates, 10g fat

Ingredients

- 90g // 3¼oz bag salad leaves
- Handful black olives, roughly chopped
- 1 tbsp capers, drained
- 2 x 120g // 4¼oz cans sardines in tomato sauce, drained and sauce reserved
- 1 tbsp olive oil
- 1 tbsp red wine vinegar

Instructions

1 Divide the salad leaves between 4 plates, then sprinkle over the olives and capers.
2 Roughly break up the sardines and add to the salad.
3 Mix the tomato sauce with the oil and vinegar. Drizzle over the salad just before serving.

Pumpkin and Sausage Soup

Serves 4
Per serving: 527 calories, 33g protein, 6g carbohydrates, 41g fat

Ingredients

- 650g // 23oz fresh sausage meat
- 1 white onion, minced
- 1 red bell pepper, diced
- 1 garlic clove, minced
- 1 pinch salt
- ½ tsp dried sage
- ½ tsp dried thyme
- ½ tsp red chilli flakes (optional)
- 120ml // ½ cup pumpkin puree
- 350ml // 1½ cups chicken stock
- 120ml // ½ cup whipping cream
- 1 tbsp salted butter

Instructions

1 Use a large pan to brown the sausage, onion, and pepper on a medium to high heat.

2 When the pork is thoroughly cooked and the onions and pepper are browned (about 10 to 15 minutes), sprinkle in the seasonings and stir to mix.

3 Stir in the pumpkin, broth, and cream. Simmer uncovered on low heat for 15 to 20 minutes or until the soup has thickened.

4 Add the butter, stir well, and serve warm.

TOP TIPS

You can easily make this recipe into a heartier meal by adding sliced mushrooms to the pan with the sausage, onion, and pepper.

Roast Beef and Cheddar Plate

Serves 2
Per serving: 838 calories, 40g protein, 6g carbohydrates, 70g fat

Ingredients

- 230g // 8oz roast beef, sliced
- 140g // 5oz cheddar cheese, cut into fingers
- 1 avocado
- 6 radishes
- 1 spring onion, sliced
- 4 tbsp mayonnaise
- 1 tbsp Dijon mustard
- 55g // 2oz lettuce
- 1 tbsp olive oil
- Salt and pepper

Instructions

1 Arrange the roast beef, cheese, avocado, scallion, and radishes on a plate.
2 Serve with lettuce, olive oil, mustard, and a hearty dollop of mayonnaise.

Smoked Trout, Watercress and Beetroot Salad

Serves 4
Per serving: 436 calories, 17g protein, 7g carbohydrates, 38g fat

Ingredients

- 1 tbsp French mustard
- 150ml // ⅔oz olive oil
- 50ml // ¼oz vinegar
- 250g // 8¾oz cooked beetroot
- 2x 135g // 4¾oz packs smoked trout fillets
- 145g // 5oz watercress, large stalks removed
- 1 tbsp creamed horseradish

Instructions

1 Take an empty jam jar with a lid. Put in a pinch of salt, a good grind of pepper, plus the mustard, olive oil and vinegar. Shake and place the jar in the fridge. Any leftover dressing you have will last a few weeks.

2 Cut the beetroot into quarters and place in a bowl. Add in the creamed horseradish and 2 tbsp of the prepared dressing and stir well.

3 Remove the skin from the trout and break the fish into small pieces. Mix the watercress and the beetroot, then top with the smoked trout.

Mexican Egg Rolls

Serves 2
Per serving: 133 calories, 9g protein, 2g carbohydrates, 10g fat

Ingredients

- 1 large egg
- A little rapeseed oil for frying
- 2 tbsp tomato salsa
- About 1 tbsp fresh coriander

Instructions

1 Beat the egg with 1 tbsp water. Heat the oil in a medium non-stick frying pan. Add the egg and swirl round the base of the pan, as though you are making a pancake, and cook until set. There is no need to turn it.

2 Carefully tip the pancake onto a board. Spread the salsa onto the pancake, sprinkle with the coriander, then roll it up. It can be eaten warm or cold. You can keep the roll for 2 days in the fridge.

Crab Stuffed Avocado

Serves 4
Per serving: 204 calories, 6g protein, 2g carbohydrates, 19g fat

Ingredients

- 100g // 3½oz white crabmeat
- 1 tsp Dijon mustard
- 2 tbsp olive oil
- 2 avocados
- 1 red chilli, deseeded and chopped
- Handful basil leaves

Instructions

1   To make the crab mix, flake the crabmeat into a small bowl and mix in the mustard and oil, then season to taste. Add the basil and chilli just before serving.
2   To serve, halve and stone the avocados. Fill each cavity with a quarter of the crab mix, scatter with a few of the smaller basil leaves and eat with teaspoons.

TOP TIP

The crab mixture can be made a day ahead.

Turkey and Brie Salad Sub

Serves 1
Per serving: 496 calories, 25g protein, 6g carbohydrates, 40g fat

Ingredients

- 28g // 1oz lettuce leaves
- 85g // 3oz deli turkey, sliced
- 28g // 1oz Brie
- 55g // 2oz avocado
- 45g // 1½oz tomatoes
- 14g // ½oz spring onions, sliced thinly
- 2 tbsp mayonnaise
- Salt and pepper to taste

Instructions

1 Lay two lettuce leaves out, overlapping one another to form the base of the sub. Spread out ½ of the mayonnaise over the leaves.

2 Stack the sliced turkey, avocado, tomato, and brie onto the lettuce-leaf base.

3 Finish with the remaining mayonnaise and scatter over the spring onion. Add salt and pepper to taste and lay over the other two lettuce leaves to close off the sandwich.

Tuna and Avocado Salad

Serves 4

Per serving: 639 calories, 44g protein, 7g carbohydrates, 45g fat

Ingredients

- 650g // 24oz canned tuna in water
- 3 avocados, cut into eighths
- 85g // 3oz red bell peppers, sliced
- 55g // 2oz red onion, sliced
- 140g // 5oz cucumber, quartered
- 55g // 2oz celery, diced
- 2 tbsp lime juice
- 80ml // ⅓ cup olive oil
- Salt and pepper to taste

Instructions

1 Drain the canned tuna. Turn the tuna onto a plate, use a fork to flake it.

2 Slice the red bell pepper and red onion into thin slices. Quarter the cucumber lengthways, remove the seeds, and cut into small chunks. Halve the celery, lengthways, and then cut into small pieces. Finally, peel and de-stone the avocado and cut into eighths.

3 Arrange all the ingredients in layers on a large serving platter or individual plates.

4 Place the lime juice and olive oil in a small jar and shake well to combine. Drizzle the dressing over the salad and finish off with salt and pepper to taste.

Salmon, Avocado & Cucumber Salad

Serves 4
Per serving: 458 calories, 23g protein, 7g carbohydrates, 38g fat

Ingredients

- 4 skinless salmon fillets
- Grated zest and juice of 1 lime
- 2 tsp clear honey
- 3 tbsp olive oil, plus a little extra for the salmon
- 3 avocados
- 1 cucumber
- 400g // 14oz mixed salad leaves
- 4 tbsp chopped mint

Instructions

1 Season the salmon, then rub with a little oil.
2 Mix the lime juice, zest, honey, and olive oil together.
3 Halve, stone, peel and slice the avocados. Halve and quarter the cucumber lengthways, then cut into slices. Divide the salad, avocado and cucumber between four plates, then drizzle with half of the dressing.
4 Heat a non-stick pan over a medium heat. Add the salmon and fry for 3 to 4 minutes on each side until crisp but still moist inside. Put a salmon fillet on top of each salad and drizzle over the remaining dressing. Serve warm.

Beef Salad with Caper and Parsley Dressing

Serves 4
Per serving: 628 calories, 40g protein, 7g carbohydrates, 50g fat

Ingredients

- 500g // 17½oz your choice of green salad leaves
- 175g // 6oz cherry tomatoes
- 4-5 roasted red peppers from a jar
- 8-12 slices cooked roast beef
- 2 tbsp lemon juice
- 1 tbsp wholegrain mustard
- 1 tbsp capers
- 3 tbsp chopped parsley
- 5 tbsp olive oil

Instructions

1 Scatter the salad leaves, tomatoes, and red peppers over a platter or large plate, then arrange the beef slices on top.
2 Put all the dressing ingredients into a small bowl with some salt and pepper, then whisk vigorously with a fork until thickened.
3 Drizzle over the beef and salad to serve.

Peppered Mackerel and Pink Pickled Onion Salad

Serves 6
Per serving: 318 calories, 13g protein, 7g carbohydrates, 25g fat

Ingredients

- 240g // 8½oz peppered smoked mackerel, torn into pieces
- 100g // 3½oz bag watercress
- 250g // 8¾oz ready-cooked beetroot

- 100g // 3½oz honey-roasted mixed nuts
- 1 small red onion, very thinly sliced
- 3 tbsp sherry vinegar
- Pinch of sugar
- 4 tbsp extra virgin olive oil

Instructions

1 Mix the onion, vinegar, sugar, and a pinch of salt. Leave to pickle while you dice the beetroot and roughly chop the nuts.

2 Divide the watercress and smoked mackerel between six plates. Scatter over the beetroot and nuts, then top with a cluster of the pickled onions. Whisk the oil into the pickling vinegar, then drizzle the dressing around the outside of each plate.

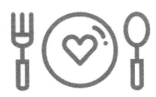

DINNER

Dinner is an important meal, and certainly no less so when following a Keto diet. Our collection of Keto dinner recipes is packed with nutrients and flavour that the whole family will love.

Creamy Sundried Tomato and Parmesan Chicken with Courgette Noodles

Serves 6
Per serving: 394 calories, 35.6g protein, 9.2g carbohydrates, 22.6g fat

Ingredients

- 1 tbsp butter

- 700g // 25oz skinless chicken thigh fillets, cut into strips

- 120g // 4oz fresh semi-dried tomato strips in oil, chopped

- 110g // 3.5oz jarred sun-dried tomatoes in oil, chopped

- 4 cloves of garlic, peeled and crushed

- 300ml // 1¼ cups cream

- 150g // 5¼oz grated parmesan cheese

- 2 large courgettes (zucchini) or squash made into noodles

Instructions

1 Heat the butter in a pan or skillet over medium to high heat. Add the chicken strips and sprinkle with salt. Pan fry until the chicken is golden brown on all sides and cooked through.

2 Add both the semi-dried and sun-dried tomatoes with 1 tablespoon of the oil from the jar (optional, but this adds extra flavour) and add the garlic. Sauté until fragrant.

3 While the chicken is browning, prepare your noodles, either with a spiraliser or using a vegetable peeler.

4 Lower the heat, add the cream and the Parmesan cheese. Simmer whilst stirring until the cheese has melted through. Sprinkle over the salt, basil, and red chilli flakes to your taste.

5 Stir through the noodles and continue to simmer until they have softened to your liking (about 5-8 minutes) and serve.

Masala Frittata and Avocado Salsa

Serves 4
Per serving: 347 calories, 16g protein, 12g carbohydrates, 25g fat

Ingredients

- 1 avocado, cubed

- 3 onions, sliced

- 8 large eggs

- 1 red chilli, deseeded and chopped

- 2 tbsp rapeseed oil

- 1 tbsp Madras paste

- 500g // 17½oz cherry tomatoes, chopped

- Small bunch of coriander, roughly chopped

- Juice of 1 lemon

Instructions

1   Heat the oil in a non-stick, ovenproof pan. Cook the sliced onions over a medium heat for around 10 minutes until they start to soften and turn golden.

2   Add the Madras paste and fry for 1 minute, then tip in half the tomatoes and half the chilli.

3   Cook until the mix thickens, and the tomatoes burst.

4   Set the grill on high. Add half the coriander to the eggs and season with salt and pepper, then pour over the spicy onion mixture.

5   Stir gently once or twice, then cook over a low heat for around 8 to 10 minutes until nearly set.

6   Transfer to the grill for a further 3 to 5 minutes until set.

7   To make the salsa, mix the avocado, remaining chilli, tomatoes, chopped onion, remaining coriander and the lemon juice together.

8   Season the salsa and serve with the frittata.

Air Fryer Chicken Thighs

Serves 4
Per serving: 213 calories, 19.3g protein, 0.9g carbohydrates, 14.2g fat

Ingredients

- 4 chicken thighs, boneless
- 2 tsp olive oil
- 1 tsp smoked paprika
- ¾ tsp garlic powder
- ½ tsp salt
- ½ tsp cracked black pepper

Instructions

1 Preheat the air fryer to 200C // 400F.
2 Pat the chicken dry and brush the skin of each thigh with oil. Place the chicken thighs on a plate.
3 Mix the paprika, garlic powder, salt, and pepper in a bowl. Sprinkle half the seasoning over the chicken thighs. Turn the chicken over and sprinkle the rest of the seasoning on top.
4 Place the chicken thighs in the air fryer, skin-side up.
5 Cook for 18 minutes until the chicken is brown and juices run clear.

Cauliflower Casserole

Serves 2
Per serving: 29 calories, 2.5g protein, 1.3g carbohydrates, 1.5g fat

Ingredients

- ½ head cauliflower, cut into florets
- 150g // 5¼oz grated cheddar cheese
- 120ml // ½ cup whipping cream
- Pinch of salt and pepper to taste

Instructions

1 Preheat the oven to 200C // 400F.
2 Bring a large pot of slightly salted water to a boil and cook the cauliflower until tender but firm to the bite, about 10 minutes, then drain the cauliflower.
3 Combine the cheddar cheese, cream, salt, and pepper in a large bowl. Arrange the cauliflower in a casserole dish and cover with the cheese mixture.
4 Bake in the oven until the cheese is bubbly and golden brown, about 25 minutes.

White Chicken Chilli

Serves 8
Per serving: 591 calories, 31.8g protein, 5.2g carbohydrates, 49.6g fat

Ingredients

- 1 tbsp oil
- 125g // 4½oz butter
- 900g // 31¾oz chicken breasts
- 1¼tsp chilli powder
- 175ml // ¾ cup chicken broth
- 475ml // 2 cups whipping cream
- 115g // 4oz cream cheese
- 150g // 5¼oz grated Monterey Jack cheese
- 2 x 230g // 4oz cans of chopped green chillies
- 1½tbsp onion powder
- 2 tsp cumin
- 1 tsp hot sauce
- Salt and pepper to taste

Instructions

1 Heat a large pan over a medium-high heat. Add the oil and 2 tablespoons of the butter.

2 Meanwhile, season the chicken with chilli powder, salt, and black pepper. Cook the chicken in the pan on 1 side for 5 minutes, resisting the urge to flip early. Turn and cook, turning occasionally to keep from burning, until no longer pink inside and the juices run clear. This should take around 10 to 15 minutes, depending on the thickness of the chicken.

3 Transfer the chicken to a plate to cool until safe to handle. Shred the chicken using your fingers and set aside.

4 Mix the remaining 6 tablespoons of butter, chicken broth, heavy cream, cream cheese, onion powder, cumin, and hot sauce together in a large, heavy pot. Season with salt and black pepper and bring to a simmer. Cook for about 5 minutes until the butter and cream cheese are melted.

5 Add the shredded chicken, Monterey Jack cheese, and green chillies to the chilli in the pot. Reduce the heat to low and cook, stirring occasionally, for 20 minutes.

Spinach and Artichoke Chicken

Serves 4
Per serving: 554 calories, 56g protein, 5.4g carbohydrates, 33.3g fat

Ingredients

- 285g // 10oz frozen spinach
- 115g // 4oz cream cheese
- 200g // 7oz (half a can) quartered artichoke hearts, drained, and chopped
- 50g // 1 ¾oz grated Parmesan cheese
- 2 tbsp mayonnaise
- ½ tsp garlic powder
- ½ tsp salt
- 680g // 24oz chicken breasts
- Salt and pepper to season
- 1 tbsp olive oil
- 100g // 3½oz mozzarella

Instructions

1 Microwave the spinach in a medium bowl until warm for around 2 to 3 minutes. Let cool slightly and squeeze to remove the moisture.

2 Return the spinach to the bowl. Mix in the cream cheese, artichoke hearts, Parmesan cheese, mayonnaise, garlic powder, and salt. Set aside.

3 Pound the chicken breasts to an even thickness that is no more than an inch thick. Season with salt and pepper.

4 Preheat the oven to 190C // 375F.

5 Heat the oil in a large pan over medium to high heat. Brown the chicken in the hot oil, working in batches.

6 Place the chicken breasts in a large baking dish. Spread the spinach and artichoke mixture on top.

7 Bake for around 20 minutes until the chicken is no longer pink inside and any juices run clear.

8 Top the breasts with the mozzarella cheese and continue baking until the cheese has melted.

Bacon and Avocado Frittata

Serves 4
Per serving: 467 calories, 22g protein, 7g carbohydrates, 38g fat

Ingredients

- 8 rashers smoked bacon
- 3 tbsp extra-virgin olive oil
- 6 eggs
- 1 large avocado, cut into slices
- 1 red chilli, finely chopped
- 1 tsp Dijon mustard
- 2 tsp red wine vinegar
- 200g // 7oz salad leaves of your choice
- 12 plum or cherry tomatoes

Instructions

1 Heat an ovenproof pan and fry the bacon on a high heat until crisp.
2 Chop the rashers roughly. Place the bacon on kitchen paper to drain, and carefully clean the pan.
3 Heat the grill, and warm 1 tbsp olive oil in the clean pan. Season and beat the eggs, stir in half of the bacon, and tip into the pan.
4 Cook on a low heat for 8 minutes until nearly set. Arrange the avocado slices and remainder of the bacon on top of the frittata, and grill for around 4 minutes until firm.
5 Mix the leftover oil, chilli, vinegar, mustard in a bowl. Season to taste.
6 Toss the salad and tomatoes in the dressing and serve with the frittata.

Tarragon, Mushroom & Sausage Frittata

Serves 2
Per serving: 433 calories, 25g protein, 8g carbohydrates, 32g fat

Ingredients

- 1 tbsp olive oil
- 200g // 7oz chestnut mushrooms, sliced
- 2 pork sausages
- 1 garlic clove, crushed
- 100g // 3½oz fine asparagus
- 3 large eggs
- 2 tbsp half-fat soured cream
- 1 tbsp wholegrain mustard
- 1 tbsp chopped tarragon
- Mixed rocket salad, to serve (optional)

Instructions

1   Heat the grill to high. Heat the oil in a medium-sized, non-stick frying pan. Add the mushrooms and fry over a high heat for 3 minutes. Squeeze the sausage meat out of the skins and shape into nuggets, add to the pan and fry for a further 5 minutes until golden brown. Add the garlic and asparagus and cook for another 1 minute.

2   Whisk the eggs, soured cream, mustard, and tarragon in a jug. Season well, then pour the egg mixture into the pan. Cook for 3 to 4 minutes, then grill for a further 1 to 2 minutes or until the top has just set with a slight wobble in the middle. Serve with the salad leaves if you like.

Asparagus, Pea & Feta Frittata

Serves 2
Per serving: 309 calories, 18g protein, 8g carbohydrates, 23g fat

Ingredients

- 1 tbsp olive oil
- ½ bunch asparagus, trimmed and cut into 5cm pieces
- 100g // 3½oz frozen peas
- 50g // 1¾oz feta
- 1 tbsp fresh mint
- 3 eggs
- 1 tbsp balsamic glaze or vinegar
- Handful of cherry or baby plum tomatoes
- Your choice of green salad to serve

Instructions

1   Heat the oven to 180C // 350F. Put the olive oil in a small ovenproof dish. Place in the oven to heat for 2 or 3 minutes.

2   Add the asparagus and peas to the oil and gently toss to coat. Bake for a further 2 minutes, then remove from the oven and crumble over the feta.

3   Whilst the vegetables bake, beat the eggs with the mint and season well. Remove the vegetables from the oven and pour over the egg mixture. Bake for 15 minutes until the eggs are cooked.

4   Quarter the tomatoes, and drizzle with the balsamic vinegar or glaze. Serve with the frittata and salad.

Prawn, Coconut and Tomato Curry

Serves 4
Per serving: 335 calories, 19g protein, 7g carbohydrates, 26g fat

Ingredients

- 2 tbsp vegetable oil
- 1 medium onion, thinly sliced
- 2 garlic cloves, sliced
- 1 green chilli, deseeded and sliccd
- 3 tbsp curry paste
- 1 tbsp tomato purée
- 200ml // ¾ cup vegetable stock
- 200ml // ¾ cup coconut cream
- 350g // 12¼oz raw prawns
- Coriander sprigs and rice, to serve

Instructions

1   Heat the oil in a large frying pan. Fry the onion, garlic and half the chilli for 5 minutes or until softened. Add the curry pastc and cook for 1 minute more. Add the tomato purée, stock, and coconut cream.

2   Simmer on a medium heat for 10 minutes, then add the prawns. Cook for 3 minutes or until they turn opaque.

3   Scatter on the remaining green chillies and coriander sprigs, then serve with rice.

Lamb and Lettuce Pan Fry

Serves 4
Per serving: 465 calories, 30g protein, 3g carbohydrates, 37g fat

Ingredients

- 25g // ¾oz butter
- 4 lamb neck fillets, cut into chunks
- 2 handfuls frozen peas
- 150ml // ¾ cup chicken stock
- 3 Baby Gem lettuces, cut into quarters

Instructions

1   Heat the butter in a frying pan until sizzling, then add the lamb. Season with salt and pepper to taste, then cook for 6 to 7 minutes until browned on all sides. Scatter in the peas, pour in the stock, then bring up to a simmer and gently cook until the peas have defrosted.
2   Add the lettuce to the pan and simmer for a few minutes until just starting to wilt, but still vibrant green. Serve scooped straight from the pan.

Pizza

Serves 4
Per serving: 617 calories, 33g protein, 6g carbohydrates, 50g fat

Ingredients

Crust:

- 170g // 6oz mozzarella, shredded
- 2 tbsp cream cheese
- 85g // 3oz almond flour

Topping:

- 230g // 8oz fresh Italian-style sausage
- 1 tbsp butter
- 120ml // ½ cup tomato sauce
- ½ tsp dried oregano
- 170g // 6oz mozzarella, shredded

- 1 tsp white wine vinegar
- 1 egg
- ½ tsp salt
- Olive oil, to grease your hands

Instructions

1 Preheat the oven to 200C // 400F.
2 Heat the mozzarella and cream cheese in a non-stick pan on medium heat or in a bowl in the microwave. Stir until they melt together. Add the other ingredients and mix well.
3 Moisten your hands with olive oil and flatten the dough on parchment paper, making a circle around 8" (20 cm) in diameter. You can also use a rolling pin to flatten the dough between two sheets of parchment paper.
4 Remove the top parchment sheet (if used). Prick the crust all over with a fork and bake in the oven for 10 to 15 minutes until golden brown. Remove from the oven.
5 While the crust is baking, sauté the ground sausage meat in olive oil or butter.
6 Spread a thin layer of tomato sauce on the crust. Top the pizza with meat and plenty of cheese. Bake for 10 to 15 minutes or until the cheese has melted.
7 Sprinkle with the oregano and serve.

TOP TIP

If you have one, use a hand mixer with dough hooks.

Fried Chicken with Broccoli

Serves 2
Per serving: 484 calories, 43g protein, 5g carbohydrates, 31g fat

Ingredients

- 260g // 9oz broccoli
- 55g // 2oz butter

- 400g // 14oz boneless chicken thighs
- Salt and pepper

Instructions

1 Rinse and trim the broccoli. Cut the broccoli into smaller pieces, including the stem.

2 Heat up a generous dollop of butter in a frying pan where you can fit both the chicken and the broccoli.

3 Season the chicken and fry over medium heat for about 5 minutes per side, or until golden brown and cooked through.

4 Add more butter and put the broccoli in the same frying pan. Fry for another couple of minutes.

5 Season to taste and serve with the remaining butter.

Chilli Salmon with Tomato and Asparagus

Serves 4
Per serving: 668 calories, 34g protein, 4g carbohydrates, 57g fat

Ingredients

- 550g // 19½oz salmon

- 140g // 5oz butter

- 2 tsp sambal oelek or chilli paste

- 550g // 19½oz green asparagus

- 140g // 5oz cherry tomatoes

- 2 tbsp olive oil

- 2 tbsp almonds, flaked or chopped

- 2 tbsp fresh thyme or parsley

- Pinch of salt

Instructions

1. Start by melting the butter over a medium heat. Heat until it starts to get a nutty scent and turns a brown colour. Stir occasionally and make sure it doesn't burn. Set aside but keep warm.

2. Brush or thinly spread sambal oelek (or chilli paste) all over the salmon. If you're using chilli paste, dilute with water or oil, so it doesn't overpower the dish. Salt generously.

3. Fry for a few minutes on each side in a hot and spacious pan with a little olive oil.

4. Cut the asparagus into 3 or 4 pieces and slice the tomatoes in half. Fry for a few minutes in a pan with a little oil. Salt and pepper to taste.

5. Serve the salmon on a bed of vegetables with a few sprigs of any fresh herb, freshly roasted almonds, and a splash of browned butter.

Chicken Meatball Poppers

Makes 28 to 30 meatballs
Per meatball: 47 calories, 4.1g protein, 0.3g carbohydrates, 3.3g fat

Ingredients

- 450g // 15¾oz minced chicken
- 1 egg
- 100g // 3½oz grated parmesan
- 1 tsp garlic powder
- 1 tsp onion powder
- 1 tsp smoked paprika
- ½ tsp salt
- Handful of chopped parsley (optional)

Instructions

1 Preheat your oven to 220C // 425F. Line a baking tray with foil and lightly spray the foil with non-stick spray.

2 Add the minced chicken, parmesan cheese, egg, fresh parsley and spices to a large bowl and mix using your hands until everything is well incorporated. Using a large spoon or ice cream scoop, portion out your meatballs and place them on your baking sheet. You should get approximately 28-30 meatballs.

3 Bake for 25 minutes, remove from the oven, and dig in! Deliciously served in a dish or alone as a snack. They go perfectly with salsa or guacamole.

TOP TIP

This recipe also works well with minced turkey.

Veggie Packed BBQ Meatloaf

Serves 4
Per serving: 252 calories, 30.6g protein, 9.8g carbohydrates, 9.4g fat

Ingredients

- 1 small courgette (zucchini), grated

- 1 small carrot, grated

- 100g // 3½oz peeled pumpkin, grated

- 500g // 17½oz extra-lean pork mince

- 4 green onions, sliced

- 30g // 1oz fresh wholemeal breadcrumbs

- 1 egg

- 80g // 2¾oz BBQ sauce, plus extra to serve

- 1 tbsp no-added-salt tomato paste

Instructions

1 Preheat the oven to 200C // 380F. Lightly spray a 10cm x 18cm loaf tin with oil and line 2 long sides with baking paper, extending the paper 2cm above the edges of the pan.

2 Squeeze excess moisture from the grated vegetables and place in a large bowl. Add the mince, green onions, breadcrumbs, egg and 1 tablespoon of the BBQ sauce. Season to taste with salt and pepper.

3 Using clean hands, mix until well combined. Press the mixture into the prepared tin. Bake for 20 minutes or until the meatloaf is cooked through when tested with a skewer. Remove and drain any excess juices from the pan.

4 Carefully turn the meatloaf top side up onto a baking tray lined with baking paper. Combine the remaining BBQ sauce and tomato paste. Brush the sauce over the meatloaf. Bake for a further 10 minutes.

5 Remove from the oven and stand for 5 minutes before slicing.

Grilled Smoky Beef Burger on a Mushroom Bun

Serves 4
Per serving: 503 calories, 33.6g protein, 12.9g carbohydrates, 36.4g fat

Ingredients

- 400g // 14oz beef mince
- 2 ½ tbsp BBQ sauce
- 1tsp smoked paprika
- 1 small courgette (zucchini), grated and squeezed of excess moisture
- 4 large field mushrooms
- 1tbsp olive oil
- 1 red onion, cut into rings
- 4x 20g // ¾oz slices cheddar cheese
- 80g // 2¾oz baby rocket leaves
- 1½ tbsp tomato sauce
- 1 large avocado, mashed
- 1 tomato, sliced

Instructions

1 Using clean hands combine the mince, smoked paprika, grated courgette and 1 tablespoon of the BBQ sauce in a large bowl. Shape into four 2cm-thick patties.

2 Heat a large chargrill pan over a medium to high heat. Brush the patties and mushrooms lightly with oil. Cook the mushrooms for 4 to 5 minutes each side or until mushrooms are lightly charred and tender. Cook the burgers for 4 minutes or until the underside is lightly charred. Turn the burgers and cook for a further 2 minutes.

3 Top each burger with a slice of cheese and cook for a further 2 minutes or until the burgers are cooked through and the cheese is melted. Cook the onion rings for 2 minutes on each side or until lightly charred.

4 Meanwhile, combine the tomato sauce and remaining BBQ sauce in a small bowl.

5 To serve, top each mushroom with avocado, rocket, sliced tomato, a burger patty, and onion rings. Serve drizzled with the sauce.

Low-Carb Chicken Parmigiana

Serves 4
Per serving: 450 calories, 32.6g protein, 7.6g carbohydrates, 31.8g fat

Ingredients

- 3 tbsp olive oil
- 1 small aubergine (eggplant) cut into 1cm thick slices
- 500g // 17½oz chicken thigh fillets
- 250g // 9oz cherry tomatoes, halved
- 175g // 6¼oz tomato and basil pasta sauce
- 100g // 3½oz fresh mozzarella
- 1 tbsp lightly toasted pine nuts
- Handful of fresh basil leaves
- Mixed salad leaves to serve

Instructions

1 Heat 1 tablespoon of oil in a large non-stick frying pan over high heat. Cook the aubergine slices in two batches for 2 minutes each side or until golden, adding another tablespoon of oil for the second batch. Transfer to a plate and set aside.

2 Return the same pan to medium to high heat. Add the remaining oil and chicken and cook for 3 to 4 minutes each side or until golden and almost cooked through. Transfer to a plate and set aside. Add the tomatoes to the pan and cook, stirring, for 2 minutes or until softened. Add the pasta sauce to the pan and simmer for 2 to 3 minutes or until thick.

3 Preheat the grill on high. Return the chicken to the pan. Top each piece of chicken with 2 aubergine slices and some cheese. Simmer for 2-3 minutes, then place under the preheated grill until cheese is melted and bubbling.

4 Serve with toasted pine nuts, basil leaves, and mixed salad.

Chilli Covered Salmon with Spinach

Serves 4
Per serving: 677 calories, 39g protein, 2g carbohydrates, 56g fat

Ingredients

- 55g // 2oz butter or olive oil
- 650g // 23oz boneless salmon fillets, cut into chunks
- Salt and pepper to taste

- 120ml // ½ cup mayonnaise
- 1 tbsp sambal oelek
- 1½ tbsp grated Parmesan
- 450g // 16oz fresh spinach

Instructions

1 Pre-heat the oven to 175C // 350F.
2 Grease a baking dish with half of the butter. Season the salmon with salt and pepper, and place in the baking dish, skin-side down.
3 Mix the mayonnaise, chilli paste, and parmesan cheese and spread on the salmon filets.
4 Bake for 20 minutes, or until the salmon is opaque and flakes easily with a fork.
5 Meanwhile, sauté the spinach in the remaining butter until it's wilted, about 2 minutes. Season with salt and pepper.
6 Serve immediately with the oven-baked salmon.

Spicy Shrimp Salad

Serves 4
Per serving: 592 calories, 24g protein, 8g carbohydrates, 50g fat

Ingredients

Ginger Dressing

- 60ml // ¼ cup olive oil
- 1 tbsp minced, fresh ginger
- ½ tbsp soy sauce
- ½ garlic clove, crushed
- Salt and pepper to taste

Salad

- 1 avocado
- Juice of ½ lime
- 140g // 5oz cucumber, peeled and sliced
- 55g // 2oz baby spinach
- Sea salt to season

Shrimp

- 1 tbsp olive oil
- 1 garlic clove, crushed
- 2 tsp chilli powder
- 280g // 10oz fresh shrimp, peeled and deveined
- Salt and pepper

To Serve

- 2 tsp chopped, fresh cilantro
- 2 tbsp chopped hazelnuts or salted peanuts (optional)

Instructions

Ginger Dressing

Add all the ginger dressing ingredients to a small bowl. Using an immersion blender, mix over low speed, until combined. Set aside.

Salad

1 Slice the avocado in half and remove the pit. Using a spoon, scoop out the avocado flesh, and cut it into slices. Place in a small bowl and stir together with the lime juice.

2 Arrange the spinach, avocado, and cucumber slices on a serving platter, or large plate. Season with the sea salt and set aside.

Shrimp

1 Heat the olive oil in a medium to the sized pan, over a medium heat. Stir in the garlic and chili powder. Add the shrimp, stir to combine, and fry for a couple of minutes each side until the shrimp are pink and cooked through. Be careful not to overcook the shrimp or it may be rubbery. Pre-cooked shrimp should only be heated through for between 1 and 2 minutes. Season with salt and pepper, to taste.

2 Use a slotted spoon to place the shrimp, with some of the spicy sauce, on top of the vegetables. Sprinkle the nuts and cilantro on top, and drizzle with the ginger dressing to serve.

Pork and Green Pepper Stir Fry

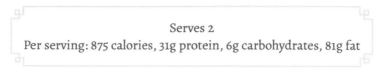

Serves 2
Per serving: 875 calories, 31g protein, 6g carbohydrates, 81g fat

Ingredients

- 110g // 4oz butter
- 300g // 10½oz pork shoulder, cut into thin slices
- 230g // 8oz green bell peppers, cut in half, seeds removed and sliced
- 30g // 1oz spring onions, chopped
- 3 tsp chilli paste
- 3 tbsp almonds
- Salt and pepper to taste

Instructions

1 Melt the butter in a frying pan or wok over medium to high heat.
2 Add the pork strips, and stir fry for a couple of minutes, or until lightly browned.
3 Add the vegetables and chilli paste, stirring for a couple of minutes, or until crisp and tender. Season with salt and pepper to taste.
4 To serving, use a slotted spoon to distribute the stir-fry to plates, sprinkle with almonds and toss to coat.

Cauliflower and Bacon Cheese Mash

Serves 4
Per serving: 399 calories, 18.8g protein, 12.2g carbohydrates, 32.2g fat

Ingredients

- 225g // 8oz bacon, diced
- 1 large cauliflower, cut into florets
- 150g // 5¼oz grated Parmesan cheese
- 4 tbsp unsalted butter, at room temperature
- 2 tbsp vegetable oil
- ½ tbsp apple cider vinegar
- Sea salt to taste

Instructions

1. Place the bacon in a large pan and cook over medium to high heat, turning occasionally, until evenly browned, around 5 to 10 minutes. Drain the bacon on paper towels, reserving the grease in the pan.

2. Place the cauliflower in a metal or silicone steamer basket inside a multi-functional pressure cooker. Add 1 cup of water to the pot. Close and lock the lid. Select the Steam function and set the timer for 4 minutes. Allow 10 to 15 minutes for the pressure to build.

3. Release the pressure carefully using the quick-release method according to the manufacturer's instructions, about 5 minutes. Unlock and remove the lid.

4. Drain the cauliflower and transfer to a deep bowl. Add the Parmesan cheese, butter, oil, vinegar, and salt. Mix with an immersion blender until smooth. Stir in the diced bacon. Add 1 to 2 tablespoons of the reserved bacon grease.

Spaghetti Squash with Bacon and Blue Cheese

Serves 2
Per serving: 339 calories, 13.5g protein, 20.6g carbohydrates, 24.3g fat

Ingredients

- 1 small squash
- 1 tbsp olive oil
- 4 slices bacon, cut into 1 cm pieces
- 110g // 4oz mushrooms, sliced
- 1 garlic clove, minced
- 100g // 3½oz baby spinach
- 60ml // ¼ cup sour cream
- 2 tbsp crumbled blue cheese

Instructions

1   Preheat the oven to 200C // 400F and line a baking sheet with foil.

2   Cut the stem off the end of the squash using a sharp knife. Cut the squash in half lengthwise and scrape out the seeds. Brush the inside with olive oil and sprinkle with salt and pepper.

3   Bake in the preheated oven until soft, about 45 minutes. Scrape the cooked flesh out into a bowl and set aside. Return the squash shells to the baking sheet.

4   Place the bacon in a large pan and cook over medium to high heat, turning occasionally, until evenly browned, 5 to 6 minutes. Drain the bacon slices on paper towels.

5   Add the mushrooms and garlic to the pan and cook for 4 to 5 minutes. Add in the cooked bacon and spinach. Stir until the spinach is wilted, 2 to 3 minutes. Add the mushroom mixture to the bowl of squash. Mix in the sour cream, salt, and pepper. Stir until the filling is evenly combined.

6   Spoon the filling back into the squash shells. Sprinkle each half with 1 tablespoon of blue cheese. Return to the oven and bake until the cheese is melted, and the squash is heated through, 4 to 5 minutes.

Avocado, Prawn and Fennel Cocktails

Serves 4
Per serving: 223 calories, 13g protein, 2g carbohydrates, 18g fat

Ingredients

- 4 tbsp extra-virgin olive oil
- 1 segmented orange, plus the juice from the trimmings
- Juice of 1 lemon
- 1 fennel bulb, trimmed, halved, and finely sliced
- 1 avocado, quartered, peeled, and sliced
- 200g // 7oz cooked king prawns
- 3 spring onions, sliced
- 55g // 2oz wild rocket

Instructions

1 Make the dressing by mixing the oil and citrus juices together in a small bowl with some salt and pepper, then set aside.

2 In a bowl, toss all the other ingredients, except the rocket, together with the orange segments and half of the dressing. Scatter the rocket leaves into 4 Martini glasses or small bowls, pile the salad into the centre, then drizzle with the remaining dressing just before serving.

DESSERT

The intricacies of the Keto diet might make it sound like you cannot enjoy your desserts at first, but that couldn't be further from the truth. Our collection of Keto dessert recipes is all as delicious as their non-Keto equivalents, just with fewer carbohydrates.

Brownie Bombs

Makes 16
Per brownie bomb: 118 calories, 5g protein, 2g carbohydrates, 9g fat

Ingredients

- 250g // 9oz smooth peanut butter
- 65g // 2¼oz cocoa powder
- 4-5 tbsp sweetener
- ¼ tsp salt
- 2 tbsp coconut oil (optional)

Instructions

1. Simply add all the ingredients to a food processor, scraping down the sides occasionally, until combined into a smooth dough.
2. If you're using a liquid sweetener and/or coconut oil, you will need to refrigerate the dough in the fridge until the mixture is firm enough to scoop into balls with a small ice cream scoop or spoon. Roll into balls of your desired size and enjoy!

Pumpkin Cheesecake

Serves 16
Per serving: 245 calories, 8.6g protein, 8.5g carbohydrates, 20.5g fat

Ingredients

- 225g // 8oz low-fat cream cheese (at room temperature)
- 4 tbsp granular sweetener
- 425g // 15oz pumpkin puree
- 1 tsp vanilla extract
- 1 tsp ground cinnamon
- ½ tsp ground ginger
- ¼ tsp ground cloves
- ¼ tsp salt
- 3 eggs

Instructions

1   Preheat the oven to 175C // 350F.

2   Pulse the almonds and pecans together in a food processor until ground, but not paste-like. Add the sweetener and butter then pulse to combine. Press the mixture into the bottom of a 9-inch springform pan.

3   Bake in the preheated oven until the crust is golden brown, about 10 minutes. Let cool for a further 10 minutes.

4   Blend the cream cheese and sweetener in a food processor or with an electric mixer until smooth, 2 to 3 minutes. Mix in the pumpkin, vanilla extract, cinnamon, ginger, cloves, and salt until smooth, about 2 minutes more. Add in the eggs one at a time, mixing thoroughly after each addition. Pour the batter into the prepared crust.

5   Bake in the preheated oven until just set in the centre, or when the filling jiggles but does not run, 45 to 50 minutes. Let cool completely, for around 30 minutes. Run a knife around the edge of the cheesecake, cover, and refrigerate for at least 4 hours until ready to serve.

No-Churn Keto Ice Cream

Serves 3
Per serving: 291 calories, 1.6g protein, 3.2g carbohydrates, 29.4g fat

Ingredients

- 230ml // 1 cup whipping cream
- 2 tbsp powdered sweetener
- 1 tbsp vodka
- 1 tsp vanilla extract
- ¼ tsp xanthan gum
- 1 pinch salt

Instructions

1 Combine the cream, sweetener, vodka, vanilla extract, xanthan gum, and salt in a wide-mouth pint-sized jar. Blend the cream mixture with an immersion blender in an up-and-down motion until the cream has thickened and soft peaks have formed, 60 to 75 seconds.

2 Cover the jar and place in the freezer for 3 to 4 hours, stirring every 30 to 40 minutes.

Quick Chocolate Mousse

Serves 2
Per serving: 373 calories, 5.4g protein, 6.9g carbohydrates, 37.6g fat

Ingredients

- 85g // 3oz cream cheese, softened
- 115ml // ½ cup whipping cream
- 1 tsp vanilla extract
- 2 tbsp powdered sweetener
- 2 tbsp cocoa powder
- 1 pinch salt

Instructions

1 Place the cream cheese in a large bowl and beat using an electric mixer until light and fluffy.
2 Turn the mixer to low speed and slowly add heavy cream and vanilla extract. Add the sweetener, cocoa powder, and salt, mixing until well incorporated.
3 Turn the mixer to high, and mix until light and fluffy, 1 to 2 minutes more.
4 Serve immediately or refrigerate for later.

Angel Food Cake

Serves 12
Per serving: 160 calories, 12g protein, 2g carbohydrates, 11g fat

Ingredients

- 75g // 2⅔oz almond flour

- 100g // 3½oz whey protein powder

- 1 tsp baking powder

- ¼ tsp salt

- 12 large egg whites

- 1 tsp cream of tartar or lemon juice

- 130g // 4½oz powdered erythritol, or other calorie-free icing sugar substitute

- 2 tsp vanilla extract

- 130g // 4⅓oz fresh raspberries

- 240ml // 1 cup whipping cream

Instructions

1 Preheat the oven to 160C // 325F. Prepare a cake pan (16 cup // 4 litre) or deep sheet tray by lining it with baking paper. Do not grease the pan.

2 Use a sifter or wire sieve to sift the almond flour, whey protein isolate, baking powder, and salt into a medium-sized bowl. Sift all ingredients together a second time and set aside.

3 In a separate bowl, use a hand mixer or stand mixer to whip the egg whites and cream of tartar until frothy. As the whites begin to take shape, sprinkle in the sweetener while continuing to beat the egg whites. After the sweetener is added, pour in the vanilla extract. Whip until stiff peaks form.

4 Add about one-third of the sifted ingredients to the egg whites and gently fold the dry ingredients into the egg whites. Repeat until all the dry ingredients are added. Fold the ingredients carefully so that the egg whites do not deflate.

5 Place the batter into the prepared pan and gently smooth the top until even.

6 Bake for 35-40 minutes or until the top is browned and springy to the touch. Let cool 15-20 minutes before inverting the cake from the pan. The cake may deflate slightly as it cools. A serrated knife will make cutting the cake easier.

7 Mash the raspberries with a fork in a bowl. Add more sweetener if desired depending on how sweet the raspberries are. Serve the angel food cake with whipping cream and the raspberry purée.

Cinnamon Rolls

Serves 12
Per serving: 183 calories, 6g protein, 1g carbohydrates, 17g fat

Ingredients

- 170g // 6oz mozzarella cheese, shredded

- 2 tbsp cream cheese

- 1 egg

- 110g // 3¾oz almond flour

- 96g // 3½oz powdered erythritol, or other calorie-free icing sugar substitute divided into three portions of 32g

- 2 tbsp coconut flour

- 1 tsp white wine vinegar

- ½ tsp baking soda

- 110g // 3¾oz butter, softened

- 1 tbsp ground cinnamon

Instructions

1 Preheat the oven to 185C // 365F.

2 Heat the mozzarella and cream cheese in a non-stick pan over a medium heat or in a bowl in the microwave. Stir until they melt together.

3 Add the egg, almond flour, coconut flour, white wine vinegar, baking soda and a third of the powdered erythritol and mix well to make a dough.

4 Roll out the dough between two pieces of parchment paper with a rolling pin to a square shape about 12 x 10" (30 cm x 26 cm) that's about 0.1 " (3 mm) thick. Remove the parchment paper that's on top.

5 Mix the cinnamon, a third of the erythritol, and butter in a bowl.

6 Spread the butter mixture carefully on top of the dough with a spatula.

7 Roll up the dough tightly into a log using parchment paper. Put the log in the fridge for about 20 minutes to firm up so the rolls will keep their shape when cutting.

8 Cut the log into 12 pieces with a sharp knife. Put them in a baking dish (that is big enough just to fit all the buns) lined with parchment paper or into individual cupcake cases. Bake in the oven for about 10-12 minutes or until golden. Let them cool.

9 Mix the remaining powdered erythritol with 1½ tbsp water with a small spoon in a bowl or glass. Drizzle the cinnamon rolls with the icing and let the icing harden for a couple of minutes before serving.

Egg Custard Tarts

Serves 8
Per serving: 496 calories, 10g protein, 4g carbohydrates, 48g fat

Ingredients

Crust:

- 230g // 8oz almond flour
- 4 tbsp granulated erythritol, or other sugar substitute
- ¼ tsp salt
- 85g // 3oz coconut oil, melted
- 1 egg

Custard:

- 425ml // 1¾ cups coconut cream
- ¼ tsp salt
- 3 tbsp granulated erythritol, or other sugar substitute
- 2 tsp vanilla extract
- ½ tbsp unflavoured powdered gelatine
- 2 tbsp water
- 6 egg yolks

Instructions

1 Preheat the oven to 175C // 350F.

2 Mix all the crust ingredients together in a mixing bowl.

3 Divide the crust mixture equally between individual 4" (10 cm) tart pans or in a 9" (23 cm) pie pan, preferably with a removable bottom. Press the crust mixture into the pan and pan sides, with the back of a dessert spoon, or using your fingers. Create a nice angle at the bottom of the tart base and prick all over the base with a fork.

4 Bake for 10-12 minutes, or until it turns a light, golden brown. Remove from the oven, and cool completely.

5 For the custard, first place the coconut cream, salt, erythritol, and vanilla in a medium-sized saucepan. Let it simmer for about 10 minutes. Remove from the heat.

6 Sprinkle the gelatine powder over the cold water and let bloom for 3 minutes.

7 In a separate bowl, beat the egg yolks until creamy with a mixer. Very slowly, pour the hot coconut cream into the eggs, whisking continuously, until well blended and smooth.

8 Pour everything back to the saucepan and return it to the stove over low heat. Add the gelatine, and whisk for 5 minutes, or until it has dissolved, and the mixture has slightly thickened.

9 If you notice any lumps in the custard, strain it through a sieve. Spoon the custard into the tart shells and refrigerate for at least two hours, or until set.

10 Leave to cool before serving.

Vanilla Mason Jar Ice Cream

Serves 1
Per serving: 497 calories, 6g protein, 4g carbohydrates, 47g fat

Ingredients

- 120ml // ½ cup whipping cream
- 1 egg yolk
- 1 tbsp powdered sweetener
- ½ tsp vanilla extract

Instructions

1 Add all the ingredients into a portion sized mason jar, or similar glass jar with a lid.
2 Seal the lid and shake vigorously for a minimum of 5 minutes.
3 Place the jar in the freezer, and chill for at least three hours.

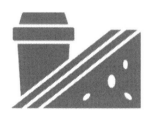

MORGAN PARKINS

SNACKS

When it comes to snacking on a Keto diet, you want to turn to things like eggs, full-fat cheese, avocados, low-carb nuts, and seeds.

Whilst a full-fat Keto diet should help you cut down on snacking, there are still going to be days where you are hungry in between meals. For those times, you want our quick and easy Keto snack recipes.

Chilli Avocado

Serves 1
Per serving: 102 calories, 1g protein, 1g carbohydrates, 10g fat

Ingredients

- ½ small avocado
- ¼ tsp chilli flakes
- Juice of ¼ lime

Instructions

Sprinkle the avocado with the chilli flakes, lime juice and a little black pepper, and eat with a spoon.

Cheese and Bacon Balls

Serves 8
Per serving: 283 calories, 11g protein, 2g carbohydrates, 26g fat

Ingredients

- 140g // 5oz bacon
- 1 tbsp butter
- 140g // 5oz cream cheese
- 140g // 5oz cheddar cheese
- 55g // 2oz butter, at room temperature
- ½ tsp pepper (optional)
- ½ tsp chilli flakes (optional)

Instructions

1 Fry the bacon in butter until golden brown. Remove from the pan and let cool completely on paper towels.
2 Crumble or chop the bacon into small pieces and place in a medium-sized bowl.
3 In a bigger bowl, mix the grease left over from frying the bacon with all the remaining ingredients by hand, or with an electric hand mixer.
4 Place the big bowl in the fridge for 15 minutes to set.
5 Shape into 24 walnut-sized balls. Roll them in the crumbled bacon and serve.

Colourful Devilled Eggs

Serves 6
Per serving: 275 calories, 13g protein, 2g carbohydrates, 24g fat

Ingredients

- 12 large eggs
- ¼ tsp salt
- 120ml // ½ cup mayonnaise
- 2 tsp Dijon mustard
- ½ tsp white pepper
- 1 tsp garlic powder
- ½ tsp turmeric
- 2 tbsp finely chopped cilantro or parsley
- 2 tbsp baby spinach, finely chopped
- 2 tbsp canned beets, mashed
- ½ tsp cider vinegar

Instructions

1 Bring a large pot of water to a rapid boil. With a large spoon, slowly add the eggs to the water one at a time. Boil for 10 minutes, then quickly drain the water from the pot and fill with cold water and ice. Let the eggs cool for 2 minutes in ice water before peeling.

2 Carefully cut your eggs in half and remove the yolks. Combine all the yolks in a large bowl with salt, mayonnaise, mustard, pepper, and garlic powder. Mix until smooth.

3 Distribute the yolk mix into three smaller bowls. To make the yellow eggs, add the turmeric to one bowl and mix until smooth then spoon the mix into 8 of the egg white shells.

4 To make the green eggs, mix the spinach and herbs into another small bowl of yolk mix. Use an immersion blender to mix well until the mix turns green. Use a clean spoon to scoop the green mix into 8 egg white shells.

5 To make the pink eggs, mix the mashed beets and vinegar into the last bowl of yolk mix. Clean the immersion blender and use it to mix until smooth. Use a spoon to scoop filling into 8 egg white shells.

6 Serve right away or set in the fridge on a tray until time to serve.

Crispy Chicken Skin

Serves 4
Per serving: 277 calories, 6g protein, 1g carbohydrates, 28g fat

Ingredients

- 250g // 9oz chicken skin
- ½ tsp paprika
- ½ tsp garlic powder
- ½ tsp salt
- ¼ tsp ground black pepper

Instructions

1 Preheat the oven to 200C // 400F.
2 Place the chicken skin pieces on a baking tray and sprinkle with the seasoning.
3 Bake in the oven for 15 minutes or until crispy.

Parmesan Chips

Serves 2
Per serving: 263 calories, 17g protein, 2g carbohydrates, 19g fat

Ingredients

- 60g // 2oz shredded Parmesan cheese
- 1 tbsp chia seeds
- 2 tbsp whole flaxseeds
- 2 ½ tbsp pumpkin seeds

Instructions

1 Preheat the oven to 180C // 350F.
2 Line a tray with baking paper.
3 Mix the cheese and seeds in a bowl.
4 Spoon small mounds of the mixture onto the baking sheet, leaving some space between them. Do not flatten the mounds. Bake for 8 to 10 minutes, checking often. The chips should be light brown, but certainly not dark brown.
5 Remove from the oven and let cool before removing the chips from the paper and serving.

Spicy Ranch Cauliflower Crackers

Makes 18 crackers
Per cracker: 29 calories, 2.5g protein, 1.3g carbohydrates, 1.5g fat

Ingredients

- 340g // 12oz frozen riced cauliflower
- 1 egg
- 1 tbsp dry ranch salad dressing mix
- ¼ tsp cayenne pepper, or more to taste
- 150g // 5¼oz grated Parmesan cheese

Instructions

1   Place the riced cauliflower in a microwave-safe bowl. Microwave, covered, for 3 to 4 minutes. Transfer to a cheesecloth-lined strainer and allow to cool for 15 minutes. Squeeze the moisture out of the cooled riced cauliflower.

2   Preheat the oven to 220C // 425F and line a baking tray with baking paper.

3   Combine the riced cauliflower, egg, ranch mix, and cayenne pepper in a bowl and mix well. Stir in the Parmesan cheese until incorporated.

4   Drop the mixture with a small cookie scoop onto the prepared cookie sheet and flatten with a small rolling pin, a cup, or your hand to approximately 1/16-inch thickness. The thinner the dough, the crispier the cracker.

5   Bake the crackers in the preheated oven for 10 minutes, flip, and bake for an additional 10 minutes. Cool on a wire rack.

BONUS – SAMPLE MEAL PLAN

To help you get started with a Keto diet and what it could look like each day, here's a sample meal plan:

Monday

Breakfast: Egg muffins
Lunch: Chicken salad with feta and olives
Dinner: Salmon with asparagus cooked in butter

Tuesday

Breakfast: Tomato, basil, and spinach omelette
Lunch: Chicken salad with feta and olives
Dinner: Vegetarian meatloaf

Wednesday

Breakfast: Scrambled eggs
Lunch: Avocado salad
Dinner: Fried chicken with broccoli

Thursday

Breakfast: Tomato baked eggs

Lunch: Mediterranean sardine salad

Dinner: Spicy shrimp salad

Friday

Breakfast: Bacon and egg baked avocado

Lunch: Roast beef and cheddar plate

Dinner: Pork and green pepper stir fry

Saturday

Breakfast: High protein breakfast bowl

Lunch: Smoked trout, watercress, and beetroot salad

Dinner: Spaghetti squash with bacon and blue cheese

Sunday

Breakfast: Breakfast wrap

Lunch: Pumpkin and sausage soup

Dinner: Masala frittata with avocado salad

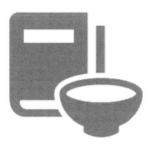

DISCLAIMER

This book contains opinions and ideas of the author and is meant to teach the reader informative and helpful knowledge while due care should be taken by the user in the application of the information provided. The instructions and strategies are possibly not right for every reader and there is no guarantee that they work for everyone. Using this book and implementing the information/ recipes therein contained is explicitly your own responsibility and risk. This work with all its contents, does not guarantee correctness, completion, quality or correctness of the provided information. Misinformation or misprints cannot be completely eliminated.

Printed in Great Britain
by Amazon